LEWY BODY DEMENTIA

Information for Patients, Families, and Professionals

LEARN ABOUT:

- Dementia with Lewy bodies
- Parkinson's disease dementia

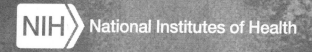

National Institute on Aging
National Institute of Neurological Disorders and Stroke

CONTENTS

Introduction

Lewy body dementia (LBD) is a complex and challenging brain disorder. It is complex because it affects many parts of the brain in ways that scientists are trying to understand more fully. It is challenging because its many possible symptoms make it hard to do everyday tasks that once came easily.

Although less known than its "cousins" Alzheimer's disease and Parkinson's disease, LBD is not a rare disorder. More than 1 million Americans, most of them older adults, are affected by its disabling changes in the ability to think and move.

As researchers seek better ways to treat LBD—and ultimately to find a cure—people with LBD and their families struggle day to day to get an accurate diagnosis, find the best treatment, and manage at home.

This booklet is meant to help people with LBD, their families, and professionals learn more about the disease and resources for coping. It explains what is known about the different types of LBD and how they are diagnosed. Most importantly, it describes how to treat and manage this difficult disease, with practical advice for both people with LBD and their caregivers. A list of resources begins on page 37.

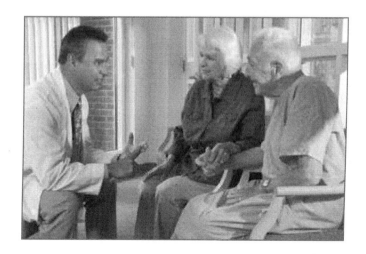

The Basics of Lewy Body Dementia

LBD is a disease associated with abnormal deposits of a protein called alpha-synuclein in the brain. These deposits, called Lewy bodies, affect chemicals in the brain whose changes, in turn, can lead to problems with thinking, movement, behavior, and mood. LBD is one of the most common causes of dementia, after Alzheimer's disease and vascular disease.

Dementia is a severe loss of thinking abilities that interferes with a person's capacity to perform daily activities such as household tasks, personal care, and handling finances. Dementia has many possible causes, including stroke, brain tumor, depression, and vitamin deficiency, as well as disorders such as LBD, Parkinson's, and Alzheimer's.

Diagnosing LBD can be challenging for a number of reasons. Early LBD symptoms are often confused with similar symptoms found in other brain diseases like Alzheimer's. Also, LBD can occur alone or along with Alzheimer's or Parkinson's disease.

There are two types of LBD—*dementia with Lewy bodies* and *Parkinson's disease dementia*. The earliest signs of these two diseases differ but reflect the same biological changes in the brain. Over time, people with dementia with Lewy bodies or Parkinson's disease dementia may develop similar symptoms.

Who Is Affected by LBD?

LBD affects more than 1 million individuals in the United States. LBD typically begins at age 50 or older, although sometimes younger people have it. LBD appears to affect slightly more men than women.

LBD is a progressive disease, meaning symptoms start slowly and worsen over time. The disease lasts an average of 5 to 7 years from the time of diagnosis to death, but the time span can range from 2 to 20 years. How

Understanding Terms

The terms used to describe Lewy body dementia (LBD) can be confusing. Doctors and researchers may use different terms to describe the same condition. In this booklet, the term *Lewy body dementia* is used to describe all dementias whose primary cause is abnormal deposits of Lewy bodies in the brain.

The two types of LBD are:

- *dementia with Lewy bodies*, in which cognitive (thinking) symptoms appear within a year of movement problems

- *Parkinson's disease dementia*, in which cognitive symptoms develop more than a year after the onset of movement problems

As LBD progresses, symptoms of both types of LBD are very similar.

quickly symptoms develop and change varies greatly from person to person, depending on overall health, age, and severity of symptoms.

In the early stages of LBD, usually before a diagnosis is made, symptoms can be mild, and people can function fairly normally. As the disease advances, people with LBD require more and more help due to a decline in thinking and movement abilities. In the later stages of the disease, they may depend entirely on others for assistance and care.

Some LBD symptoms may respond to treatment for a period of time. Currently, there is no cure for the disease. Research is improving our understanding of this challenging condition, and advances in science may one day lead to better diagnosis, improved care, and new treatments.

What Are Lewy Bodies?

Lewy bodies are named for Dr. Friederich Lewy, a German neurologist. In 1912, he discovered abnormal protein deposits that disrupt the brain's normal functioning in people with Parkinson's disease. These abnormal deposits are now called "Lewy bodies."

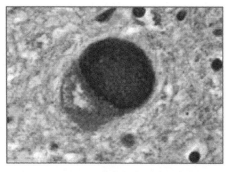

Microscopic image of a Lewy body.
Courtesy of Carol F. Lippa, MD, Drexel University College of Medicine.

Lewy bodies are made of a protein called alpha-synuclein. In the healthy brain, alpha-synuclein plays a number of important roles in neurons (nerve cells) in the brain, especially at synapses, where brain cells communicate with each other. In LBD, alpha-synuclein forms into clumps inside neurons, starting in particular regions of the brain. This process causes neurons to work less effectively and, eventually, to die. The activities of brain chemicals important to brain function are also affected. The result is widespread damage to certain parts of the brain and a decline in abilities affected by those brain regions.

Lewy bodies affect several different brain regions in LBD:

- the cerebral cortex, which controls many functions, including information processing, perception, thought, and language

- the limbic cortex, which plays a major role in emotions and behavior

- the hippocampus, which is essential to forming new memories

- the midbrain, including the substantia nigra, which is involved in movement

- the brain stem, which is important in regulating sleep and maintaining alertness

- brain regions important in recognizing smells (olfactory pathways)

Types of Lewy Body Dementia

Lewy body dementia includes two related conditions—dementia with Lewy bodies and Parkinson's disease dementia. The difference between them lies largely in the timing of cognitive (thinking) and movement symptoms. In dementia with Lewy bodies, cognitive symptoms are noted within a year of parkinsonism, any condition that involves the types of movement changes, such as tremor or muscle stiffness, seen in Parkinson's disease. In Parkinson's disease dementia, movement symptoms are pronounced in the early stages, with cognitive symptoms developing years later.

Dementia with Lewy Bodies

People with dementia with Lewy bodies have a decline in thinking ability that may look somewhat like Alzheimer's disease. But over time they also develop movement and other distinctive symptoms that suggest dementia with Lewy bodies. Symptoms that distinguish this form of dementia from others may include:

- visual hallucinations early in the course of dementia

- fluctuations in cognitive ability, attention, and alertness

- slowness of movement, difficulty walking, or rigidity (parkinsonism)

- sensitivity to medications used to treat hallucinations

Not-so-sweet dreams

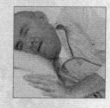

In his mid-sixties, Bruce started having some mild confusion and vivid dreams that he physically acted out by thrashing around and even falling out of bed. His neurologist diagnosed REM sleep behavior disorder and mild cognitive changes. Two years later, Bruce's confusion had progressed to dementia, and he had slowness of movement. He was no longer able to live alone in his own home. His neurologist referred him for neuropsychological testing and, based on the results, changed his diagnosis to dementia with Lewy bodies.

- REM sleep behavior disorder, in which people physically act out their dreams by yelling, flailing, punching bed partners, and falling out of bed

- more trouble with complex mental activities, such as multitasking, problem solving, and analytical thinking, than with memory

Parkinson's Disease Dementia

This type of LBD starts as a movement disorder, with symptoms such as slowed movement, muscle stiffness, tremor, and a shuffling walk. These symptoms are consistent with a diagnosis of Parkinson's disease. Later on, cognitive symptoms of dementia and changes in mood and behavior may arise.

Not all people with Parkinson's develop dementia, and it is difficult to predict who will. Being diagnosed with Parkinson's late in life is a risk factor for Parkinson's disease dementia.

Parkinson's progresses

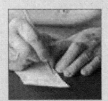

Betty is retired from the high school food-services department and is devoted to her family, especially her three granddaughters. At age 73, Betty developed a mild tremor in one hand, cramped handwriting, a shuffling gait, and a stooped posture. She was diagnosed with Parkinson's disease. When she started having hallucinations 3 years later, her children became alarmed. Betty soon started having problems with confusion and visual-spatial orientation. She was diagnosed with Parkinson's disease dementia.

Causes and Risk Factors

The precise cause of LBD is unknown, but scientists are learning more about its biology and genetics. For example, they know that an accumulation of Lewy bodies is associated with a loss of certain neurons in the brain that produce two important neurotransmitters, chemicals that act as messengers between brain cells. One of these messengers, acetylcholine, is 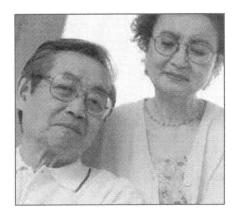 important for memory and learning. The other, dopamine, plays an important role in behavior, cognition, movement, motivation, sleep, and mood.

Scientists are also learning about risk factors for LBD. Age is considered the greatest risk factor. Most people who develop the disorder are over age 50.

Other known risk factors for LBD include the following:

* **Diseases and health conditions**—Certain diseases and health conditions, particularly Parkinson's disease and REM sleep behavior disorder, are linked to a higher risk of LBD.

* **Genetics**—While having a family member with LBD may increase a person's risk, LBD is not normally considered a genetic disease. A small percentage of families with dementia with Lewy bodies has a genetic association, such as a variant of the GBA gene, but in most cases, the cause is unknown. At this time, no genetic test can accurately predict whether someone will develop LBD. Future genetic research may reveal more information about causes and risk.

* **Lifestyle**—No specific lifestyle factor has been proven to increase one's risk for LBD. However, some studies suggest that a healthy lifestyle— including regular exercise, mental stimulation, and a healthy diet— might reduce the chance of developing age-associated dementias.

Common Symptoms

People with LBD may not have every LBD symptom, and the severity of symptoms can vary greatly from person to person. Throughout the course of the disease, any sudden or major change in functional ability or behavior should be reported to a doctor.

The most common symptoms include changes in cognition, movement, sleep, and behavior.

Cognitive Symptoms

LBD causes changes in thinking abilities. These changes may include:

- **Dementia**—Severe loss of thinking abilities that interferes with a person's capacity to perform daily activities. Dementia is a primary symptom in LBD and usually includes trouble with visual and spatial abilities (judging distance and depth or misidentifying objects), planning, multitasking, problem solving, and reasoning. Memory problems may not be evident at first but often arise as LBD progresses. Dementia can also include changes in mood and behavior, poor judgment, loss of initiative, confusion about time and place, and difficulty with language and numbers.

- **Cognitive fluctuations**—Unpredictable changes in concentration, attention, alertness, and wakefulness from day to day and sometimes throughout the day. A person with LBD may stare into space for periods of time, seem drowsy and lethargic, or sleep for several hours during the day despite getting enough sleep the night before. His or her flow of ideas may be disorganized, unclear, or illogical at times. The person may seem better one day, then worse the next day. These cognitive fluctuations are common in LBD but are not always easy for a doctor to identify.

Main Symptoms of Lewy Body Dementia

Symptom	Dementia with Lewy Bodies	Parkinson's Disease Dementia
Dementia	✔ Appears within a year of movement problems	✔ Appears later in the disease, after movement problems
Movement problems (parkinsonism)	✔ Appear at the same time as or after dementia	✔ Appear before dementia
Fluctuating cognition, attention, alertness	✔	✔
Visual hallucinations	✔	✔
REM sleep behavior disorder	● May develop years before other symptoms	● May develop years before other symptoms
Extreme sensitivity to antipsychotic medications	●	●
Changes in personality and mood (depression, delusions, apathy)	●	●
Changes in autonomic (involuntary) nervous system (blood pressure, bladder and bowel control)	●	●

✔ Primary symptom

● Common symptom

Source: Adapted from the Lewy Body Dementia Association, DLB and PDD Diagnostic Criteria, *www.lbda.org/node/470*

- **Hallucinations**—Seeing or hearing things that are not present. Visual hallucinations occur in up to 80 percent of people with LBD, often early on. They are typically realistic and detailed, such as images of children or animals. Auditory hallucinations are less common than visual ones but may also occur. Hallucinations that are not disruptive may not require treatment. However, if they are frightening or dangerous (for example, if the person attempts to fight a perceived intruder), then a doctor may prescribe medication.

Movement Symptoms

Some people with LBD may not experience significant movement problems for several years. Others may have them early on. At first, signs of movement problems, such as a change in handwriting, may be very mild and thus overlooked. Parkinsonism is seen early on in Parkinson's disease dementia but can also develop later on in dementia with Lewy bodies. Specific signs of parkinsonism may include:

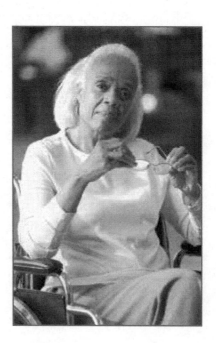

- muscle rigidity or stiffness
- shuffling gait, slow movement, or frozen stance
- tremor or shaking, most commonly at rest
- balance problems and falls
- stooped posture
- loss of coordination
- smaller handwriting than was usual for the person
- reduced facial expression
- difficulty swallowing
- a weak voice

Sleep Disorders

Sleep disorders are common in people with LBD but are often undiagnosed. A sleep specialist can play an important role on a treatment team, helping to diagnose and treat sleep disorders. Sleep-related disorders seen in people with LBD may include:

* **REM sleep behavior disorder**—A condition in which a person seems to act out dreams. It may include vivid dreaming, talking in one's sleep, violent movements, or falling out of bed. Sometimes only the bed partner of the person with LBD is aware of these symptoms. REM sleep behavior disorder appears in some people years before other LBD symptoms.

* **Excessive daytime sleepiness**—Sleeping 2 or more hours during the day.

* **Insomnia**—Difficulty falling or staying asleep, or waking up too early.

* **Restless leg syndrome**—A condition in which a person, while resting, feels the urge to move his or her legs to stop unpleasant or unusual sensations. Walking or moving usually relieves the discomfort.

Behavioral and Mood Symptoms

Changes in behavior and mood are possible in LBD. These changes may include:

* **Depression**—A persistent feeling of sadness, inability to enjoy activities, or trouble with sleeping, eating, and other normal activities.

* **Apathy**—A lack of interest in normal daily activities or events; less social interaction.

- **Anxiety**—Intense apprehension, uncertainty, or fear about a future event or situation. A person may ask the same questions over and over or be angry or fearful when a loved one is not present.

- **Agitation**—Restlessness, as seen by pacing, hand wringing, an inability to get settled, constant repeating of words or phrases, or irritability.

- **Delusions**—Strongly held false beliefs or opinions not based on evidence. For example, a person may think his or her spouse is having an affair or that relatives long dead are still living. Another delusion that may be seen in people with LBD is Capgras syndrome, in which the person believes a relative or friend has been replaced by an imposter.

- **Paranoia**—An extreme, irrational distrust of others, such as suspicion that people are taking or hiding things.

Other LBD Symptoms

People with LBD can also experience significant changes in the part of the nervous system that regulates automatic functions such as those of the heart, glands, and muscles. The person may have:

- changes in body temperature
- problems with blood pressure
- dizziness
- fainting
- frequent falls
- sensitivity to heat and cold
- sexual dysfunction
- urinary incontinence
- constipation
- a poor sense of smell

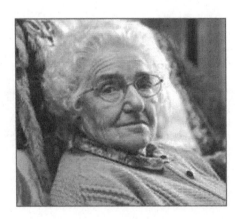

Diagnosis *I asked Dr — he never answered me.*

It's important to know which type of LBD a person has, both to tailor treatment to particular symptoms and to understand how the disease will likely progress. Clinicians and researchers use the "1-year rule" to diagnose which form of LBD a person has. If cognitive symptoms appear within a year of movement problems, the diagnosis is dementia with Lewy bodies. If cognitive problems develop more than a year after the onset of movement problems, the diagnosis is Parkinson's disease dementia.

Regardless of the initial symptoms, over time people with LBD often develop similar symptoms due to the presence of Lewy bodies in the brain. But there are some differences. For example, dementia with Lewy bodies may progress more quickly than Parkinson's disease dementia.

Dementia with Lewy bodies is often hard to diagnose because its early symptoms may resemble those of Alzheimer's, Parkinson's disease, or a psychiatric illness. As a result, it is often misdiagnosed or missed altogether. As additional symptoms appear, it is often easier to make an accurate diagnosis.

The good news is that doctors are increasingly able to diagnose LBD earlier and more accurately as researchers identify which symptoms help distinguish it from similar disorders.

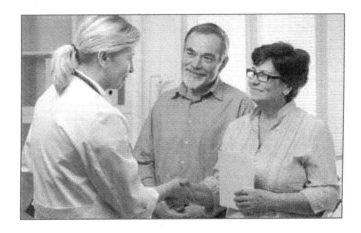

Difficult as it is, getting an accurate diagnosis of LBD early on is important so that a person:

* gets the right medical care and avoids potentially harmful treatment
* has time to plan medical care and arrange legal and financial affairs
* can build a support team to stay independent and maximize quality of life

What's going on?

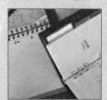

Janet, a 60-year-old executive secretary, began having trouble managing the accounting, paperwork, and other responsibilities of her job. She became increasingly irritable, and her daughter insisted she see a doctor. Janet was diagnosed with depression and stress-related problems. She was prescribed an antidepressant, but her thinking and concentration problems worsened. When she could no longer function at work, her doctor diagnosed Alzheimer's disease. A few months later, Janet developed a tremor in her right hand. She was referred to a neurologist, who finally diagnosed Lewy body dementia.

While a diagnosis of LBD can be distressing, some people are relieved to know the reason for their troubling symptoms. It is important to allow time to adjust to the news. Talking about a diagnosis can help shift the focus toward developing a care plan.

Who Can Diagnose LBD?

Many physicians and other medical professionals are not familiar with LBD, so patients may consult several doctors before receiving a diagnosis. Visiting a family doctor is often the first step for people who are experiencing changes in thinking, movement, or behavior. However, neurologists—doctors who specialize in disorders of the brain and nervous system—generally have the expertise needed to diagnose LBD. Geriatric psychiatrists, neuropsychologists, and geriatricians may also be skilled in diagnosing the condition.

If a specialist cannot be found in your community, ask the neurology department of the nearest medical school for a referral. A hospital affiliated with a medical school may also have a dementia or movement disorders clinic that provides expert evaluation. See the "Resources" section at the end of this booklet.

Tests Used to Diagnose LBD

Doctors perform physical and neurological examinations and various tests to distinguish LBD from other illnesses. An evaluation may include:

- **Medical history and examination**—A review of previous and current illnesses, medications, and current symptoms and tests of movement and memory give the doctor valuable information.

- **Medical tests**—Laboratory studies can help rule out other diseases and hormonal or vitamin deficiencies that can be associated with cognitive changes.

- **Brain imaging**—Computed tomography or magnetic resonance imaging can detect brain shrinkage or structural abnormalities and help rule out other possible causes of dementia or movement symptoms.

Magnetic resonance image of the brain.

- **Neuropsychological tests**—These tests are used to assess memory and other cognitive functions and can help identify affected brain regions.

There are no brain scans or medical tests that can definitively diagnose LBD. Currently, LBD can be diagnosed with certainty only by a brain autopsy after death.

However, researchers are studying ways to diagnose LBD more accurately in the living brain. Certain types of neuroimaging—positron emission tomography and single-photon emission computed tomography—have shown promise in detecting differences between dementia with Lewy bodies and Alzheimer's disease. These methods may help diagnose certain features of the disorder, such as dopamine deficiencies. Researchers are also investigating the use of lumbar puncture (spinal tap) to measure proteins in cerebrospinal fluid that might distinguish dementia with Lewy bodies from Alzheimer's disease and other brain disorders.

Other Helpful Information

It is important for the patient and a close family member or friend to tell the doctor about any symptoms involving thinking, movement, sleep, behavior, or mood. Also, discuss other health problems and provide a list of all current medications, including prescriptions, over-the-counter drugs, vitamins, and supplements. Certain medications can worsen LBD symptoms.

Caregivers may be reluctant to talk about a person's symptoms when that person is present. Ask to speak with the doctor privately if necessary. The more information a doctor has, the more accurate a diagnosis can be.

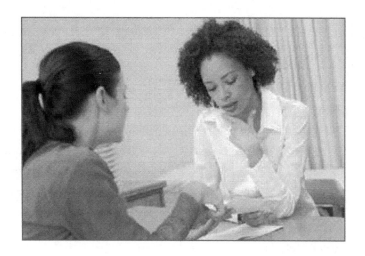

Treatment and Management

While LBD currently cannot be prevented or cured, some symptoms may respond to treatment for a period of time. A comprehensive treatment plan may involve medications, physical and other types of therapy, and counseling. Changes to make the home safer, equipment to make everyday tasks easier, and social support are also very important.

A skilled care team often can provide suggestions to help improve quality of life for both people with LBD and their caregivers.

Building a Care Team

After receiving a diagnosis, a person with LBD may benefit from seeing a neurologist who specializes in dementia and/or movement disorders. A good place to find an LBD specialist is at a dementia or movement disorders clinic in an academic medical center in your community. If such a specialist cannot be found, a general neurologist should be part of the care team. Ask a primary care physician for a referral.

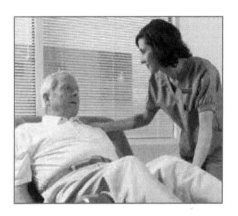

A doctor can work with other types of healthcare providers. Depending on an individual's particular symptoms, other professionals may be helpful:

- **Physical therapists** can help with movement problems through cardiovascular, strengthening, and flexibility exercises, as well as gait training and general physical fitness programs.

- **Speech therapists** may help with low voice volume, voice projection, and swallowing difficulties.

- **Occupational therapists** help identify ways to more easily carry out everyday activities, such as eating and bathing, to promote independence.

- **Music or expressive arts therapists** may provide meaningful activities that can reduce anxiety and improve well-being.

- **Mental health counselors** can help people with LBD and their families learn how to manage difficult emotions and behaviors and plan for the future.

Support groups are another valuable resource for both people with LBD and caregivers. Sharing experiences and tips with others in the same situation can help people identify practical solutions to day-to-day challenges and get emotional and social support. To find a support group near you, see the "Resources" section.

The Role of Palliative Care

The goal of palliative care (comfort care) is to improve a person's quality of life by relieving disease symptoms at any stage of illness. Palliative care can help manage LBD symptoms such as constipation, sleep disorders, and behavioral problems. Typically, a team of nurses, social workers, physical therapists, dieticians, and pharmacists works with doctors to:

- relieve troubling symptoms

- assist with medical decisions

- offer emotional and spiritual support

- coordinate care

To find a palliative medicine specialist, ask a physician or local hospital for a referral, or consult CaringInfo, a service of the National Hospice and Palliative Care Organization. Visit *www.caringinfo.org*.

Medications

Several drugs and other treatments are available to treat LBD symptoms. It is important to work with a knowledgeable health professional because certain medications can make some symptoms worse. Some symptoms can improve with nondrug treatments.

Cognitive Symptoms

Some medications used to treat Alzheimer's disease also may be used to treat the cognitive symptoms of LBD. These drugs, called cholinesterase inhibitors, act on a chemical in the brain that is important for memory and thinking. They may also improve behavioral symptoms. (See "Behavioral and Mood Problems" on page 22 for more information.)

The U.S. Food and Drug Administration (FDA) approves specific drugs for certain uses after rigorous testing and review. The FDA has approved one Alzheimer's drug, rivastigmine (Exelon®), to treat cognitive symptoms in Parkinson's disease dementia. This and other Alzheimer's drugs can have side effects such as nausea and diarrhea.

Getting treatment

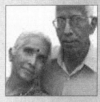

Kamar, grandfather of five, was a highly educated executive with a background in the research, development, and field testing of aircraft engines. When he retired at 67, his wife, Manjit, noticed that he had problems with complex mental activities and that his executive abilities had declined. He also had trouble with tasks involving a sequence of steps. His doctor prescribed a medication for the cognitive symptoms, which was helpful. It has been 6 years since Kamar was diagnosed, and Manjit credits the medication for helping him have a better quality of life.

Trouble with balance

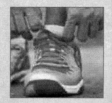

After major surgery at age 69, Cliff developed balance problems, and later his movements became stiff. Within a year, Cliff started having hallucinations and troubling side effects from anti-psychotic medications. After an initial diagnosis of parkinsonism, he soon developed cognitive problems and was diagnosed with Lewy body dementia. Cliff's balance problems increased, and many falls prompted physical and occupational therapy, where he learned to use adaptive devices and techniques. Cliff's wife, Kathy, discovered that putting his shoes on before getting him up helped improve his balance. The doctor prescribed a low dose of medication for parkinsonism, which also helped.

Movement Symptoms

LBD-related movement symptoms may be treated with a Parkinson's medication called carbidopa-levodopa (Sinemet®, Parcopa®, Stalevo®). This drug can help improve functioning by making it easier to walk, get out of bed, and move around. However, it cannot stop or reverse the progress of the disease.

Side effects of this medication can include hallucinations and other psychiatric or behavioral problems. Because of this risk, physicians may recommend not treating mild movement symptoms with medication. If prescribed, carbidopa-levodopa usually begins at a low dose and is increased gradually. Other Parkinson's medications are less commonly used in people with LBD due to a higher frequency of side effects.

A surgical procedure called deep brain stimulation, which can be very effective in treating the movement symptoms of Parkinson's disease, is not recommended for people with LBD because it can result in greater cognitive impairment.

People with LBD may benefit from physical therapy and exercise. Talk with your doctor about what physical activities are best.

Sleep Disorders

Sleep problems may increase confusion and behavioral problems in people with LBD and add to a caregiver's burden. A physician can order a sleep study to identify any underlying sleep disorders such as sleep apnea, restless leg syndrome, and REM sleep behavior disorder.

REM sleep behavior disorder, a common LBD symptom, involves acting out one's dreams, leading to lost sleep and even injuries to sleep partners. Clonazepam (Klonopin®), a drug used to control seizures and relieve panic attacks, is often effective for the disorder at very low dosages. However, it can have side effects such as dizziness, unsteadiness, and problems with thinking. Melatonin, a naturally occurring hormone used to treat insomnia, may also offer some benefit when taken alone or with clonazepam.

Sleep and dementia

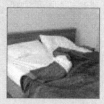

Lee started having bad nightmares in his late sixties. Later he had problems communicating and would sit for long periods of time staring out the window. His sleep problems worsened and, by age 73, were one of the most difficult symptoms of LBD. While asleep, Lee talked, his limbs jerked, and he thought his dreams were real. Upon waking, he thought he had been at work or out with friends. Medications prescribed for dementia and sleep issues helped both Lee and his wife get more rest.

Excessive daytime sleepiness is also common in LBD. If it is severe, a sleep specialist may prescribe a stimulant to help the person stay awake during the day.

Some people with LBD may have difficulty falling asleep. If trouble sleeping at night (insomnia) persists, a physician may recommend a prescription medication to promote sleep. It is important to note that treating insomnia and other sleep problems in people with LBD has not been extensively studied, and that treatments may worsen daytime sleepiness and should be used with caution.

Certain sleep problems can be addressed without medications. Increasing daytime exercise or activities and avoiding lengthy or frequent naps can promote better sleep. Avoiding alcohol, caffeine, or chocolate late in the day can help, too. Some over-the-counter medications can also affect sleep, so review all medications and supplements with a physician.

Behavioral and Mood Problems

Behavioral and mood problems in people with LBD can arise from hallucinations or delusions. They may also be a result of pain, illness, stress or anxiety, and the inability to express frustration, fear, or feeling overwhelmed. The person may resist care or lash out verbally or physically.

Caregivers must try to be patient and use a variety of strategies to handle such challenging behaviors. Some behavioral problems can be managed by making changes in the person's environment and/or treating medical conditions. Other problems may require medication.

The first step is to visit a doctor to see if a medical condition unrelated to LBD is causing the problem. Injuries, fever, urinary tract or pulmonary infections, pressure ulcers (bed sores), and constipation can worsen behavioral problems. Increased confusion can also occur.

Certain medications used to treat LBD symptoms or other diseases may also cause behavioral problems. For example, some sleep aids, pain medications, bladder control medications, and drugs used to treat LBD-related movement symptoms can cause confusion, agitation, hallucinations, and delusions. Similarly, 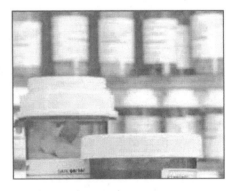 some anti-anxiety medicines can actually increase anxiety in people with LBD. Review your medications with your doctor to determine if any changes are needed.

Not all behavioral problems are caused by illness or medication. A person's surroundings—including levels of stimulation or stress, lighting, daily routines, and relationships—can lead to behavior issues. Caregivers can alter the home environment to try to minimize anxiety and stress for the person with LBD. In general, people with LBD benefit from having simple tasks, consistent

Coping with Behavioral Problems

Follow these steps in consultation with a physician to address behavioral problems:

- Rule out physical causes, like infection, pain, or other medical conditions.
- Review current prescription and over-the-counter medications.
- Look for environmental or social factors that contribute to behavioral problems.
- Consider treating with medications if necessary and watch for side effects.

schedules, regular exercise, and adequate sleep. Large crowds or overly stimulating environments can increase confusion and anxiety.

Hallucinations and delusions are among the biggest challenges for LBD caregivers. The person with LBD may not understand or accept that the hallucinations are not real and become agitated or anxious. Caregivers can help by responding to the fears expressed instead of arguing or responding factually to comments that may not be true. By tuning in to the person's emotions, caregivers can offer empathy and concern, maintain the person's dignity, and limit further tension.

Cholinesterase inhibitors may reduce hallucinations and other psychiatric symptoms of LBD. These medications may have side effects, such as nausea, and are not always effective. However, they can be a good first choice to treat behavioral symptoms. Cholinesterase inhibitors do not affect behavior immediately, so they should be considered part of a long-term strategy.

Seeing things

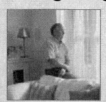

John, 58, started seeing small children outside the window who were not there. Eventually, he began talking with some of these children, whom he thought were visiting the house. These hallucinations never scared or threatened John, and they seemed to give him companionship and entertainment. His wife Linda consulted a doctor, who said that since the hallucinations were not disruptive, no medication was needed. He advised Linda not to argue with her husband about whether or not the children were there.

Antidepressants can be used to treat depression and anxiety, which are common in LBD. Two types of antidepressants, called selective serotonin reuptake inhibitors and serotonin and norepinephrine reuptake inhibitors, are often well tolerated by people with LBD.

In some cases, antipsychotic medications are necessary to treat LBD-related behavioral symptoms to improve both the quality of life and safety of the person with LBD and his or her caregiver. These types of medications must be used with caution because they can cause severe side effects and can worsen movement symptoms.

If antipsychotics are prescribed, it is very important to use the newer kind, called *atypical* antipsychotics. These medications should be used at the lowest dose possible and for the shortest time possible to control symptoms. Many LBD experts prefer quetiapine (Seroquel®) or clozapine (Clozaril®, FazaClo®) to control difficult behavioral symptoms.

Typical (or traditional) antipsychotics, such as haloperidol (Haldol®), generally should **not** be prescribed for people with LBD. They can cause dangerous side effects.

Other Treatment Considerations

LBD affects the part of the nervous system that regulates automatic actions like blood pressure and digestion. One common symptom is orthostatic hypotension, low blood pressure that can cause dizziness and fainting. Simple measures such as leg elevation, elastic stockings, and,

Warning About Antipsychotics

People with LBD may have severe reactions to or side effects from antipsychotics, medications used to treat delusions, hallucinations, or agitation. These side effects include increased confusion, worsened parkinsonism, extreme sleepiness, and low blood pressure that can result in fainting (orthostatic hypotension). Caregivers should contact the doctor if these side effects continue after a few days.

Some antipsychotics, including olanzapine (Zyprexa®) and risperidone (Risperdal®), should be avoided, if possible, because they are more likely than others to cause serious side effects.

In rare cases, a potentially deadly condition called neuroleptic malignant syndrome can occur. Symptoms of this condition include high fever, muscle rigidity, and muscle tissue breakdown that can lead to kidney failure. Report these symptoms to your doctor immediately.

Antipsychotic medications increase the risk of death in elderly people with dementia, including those with LBD. Doctors, patients, and family members must weigh the risks of antipsychotic use against the risks of physical harm and distress that may occur as a result of untreated behavioral symptoms.

when recommended by a doctor, increasing salt and fluid intake can help. If these measures are not enough, a doctor may prescribe medication.

Urinary incontinence (loss of bladder control) should be treated cautiously because certain medications used to treat this condition may worsen cognition or increase confusion. Consider seeing a urologist. Constipation can often be treated by exercise and changes in diet, though laxatives and stool softeners may be necessary.

People with LBD are often sensitive to prescription and over-the-counter medications for other medical conditions. Talk with your doctor about any side effects seen in a person with LBD.

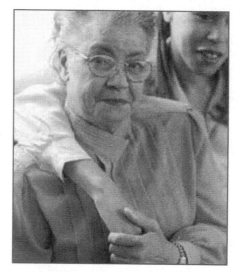

If surgery is planned and the person with LBD is told to stop taking all medications beforehand, ask the doctor to consult the person's neurologist in developing a plan for careful withdrawal. In addition, be sure to talk with the anesthesiologist in advance to discuss medication sensitivities and risks unique to LBD. People with LBD who receive certain anesthetics may become confused or delirious and have a sudden, significant decline in functional abilities, which may become permanent.

Depending on the procedure, possible alternatives to general anesthesia may include a spinal or regional block. These methods are less likely to result in confusion after surgery. Caregivers should also discuss the use of strong pain relievers after surgery, since people with LBD can become delirious if these drugs are used too freely.

Vitamins and Supplements

The use of vitamins and supplements to treat LBD symptoms has not been studied extensively and is not recommended as part of standard treatment. Vitamins and supplements can be dangerous when taken with other medicines. People with LBD should tell their doctors about every medication they take. Be sure to list prescription and over-the-counter medicines, as well as vitamins and supplements.

Advice for People Living with Lewy Body Dementia

Coping with a diagnosis of LBD and all that follows can be challenging. Getting support from family, friends, and professionals is critical to ensuring the best possible quality of life. Creating a safe environment and preparing for the future are important, too. Take time to focus on your strengths, enjoy each day, and make the most of your time with family and friends. Here are some ways to live with LBD day to day.

Getting Help

Your family and close friends are likely aware of changes in your thinking, movement, or behavior. You may want to tell others about your diagnosis so they can better understand the reason for these changes and learn more about LBD. For example, you could say that you have been diagnosed with a brain disorder called 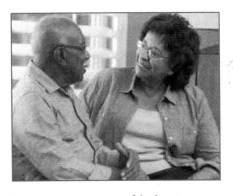 Lewy body dementia, which can affect thinking, movement, and behavior. You can say that you will need more help over time. By sharing your diagnosis with those closest to you, you can build a support team to help you manage LBD.

As LBD progresses, you will likely have more trouble managing everyday tasks such as taking medication, paying bills, and driving. You will gradually need more assistance from family members, friends, and perhaps professional caregivers. Although you may be reluctant to get help, try to let others partner with you so you can manage responsibilities together. Remember, LBD affects your loved ones, too. You can help reduce their stress when you accept their assistance.

Finding someone you can talk with about your diagnosis—a trusted friend or family member, a mental health professional, or a spiritual advisor—may be helpful. See the "Resources" section to find supportive services in your area.

Consider Safety

The changes in thinking and movement that occur with LBD require attention to safety issues. Consider these steps:

- Fill out and carry the LBD Medical Alert Wallet Card (available at *www.lbda.org/go/walletcard*) and present it any time you are hospitalized, require emergency medical care, or meet with your doctors. It contains important information about medication sensitivities.

- Consider subscribing to a medical alert service, in which you push a button on a bracelet or necklace to access 911 if you need emergency help.

- Address safety issues in your home, including areas of fall risk, poor lighting, stairs, or cluttered walkways. Think about home modifications that may be needed, such as installing grab bars in the bathroom or modifying stairs with ramps. Ask your doctor to refer you to a home health agency for a home safety evaluation.

- Talk with your doctor about LBD and driving, and have your driving skills evaluated, if needed.

Plan for Your Future

There are many ways to plan ahead. Here are some things to consider:

- If you are working, consult with a legal and financial expert about planning for disability leave or retirement. Symptoms of LBD will interfere with work performance over time, and it is essential to plan now to obtain benefits you are entitled to.

- Consult with an attorney who specializes in elder law or estate planning to help you write or update important documents, such as a living will, healthcare power of attorney, and will.

- Identify local resources for home care, meals, and other services *before* you need them so you know whom to call when the time comes.

- Explore moving to a retirement or continuing care community where activities and varying levels of care can be provided over time, as needed. Ask about staff members' experience caring for people with LBD.

Find Enjoyment Every Day

It is important to focus on living with LBD. Your attitude can help you find enjoyment in daily life. Despite the many challenges and adjustments, you can have moments of humor, tenderness, and gratitude with the people closest to you.

Make a list of events and activities you can still enjoy—then find a way to do them! For example, listening to music, exercising, or going out for a meal allows you to enjoy time with family and friends. If you can't find pleasure in daily life, consult your doctor or another healthcare professional to discuss effective ways to cope and move forward. Let your family know if you are struggling emotionally so they can offer support.

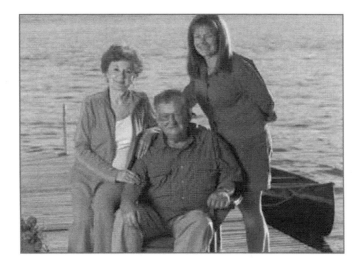

Caring for a Person with Lewy Body Dementia

As someone who is caring for a person with LBD, you will take on many different responsibilities over time. You do not have to face these responsibilities alone. Many sources of help are available, from adult day centers and respite care to online and in-person support groups.

A peaceful routine

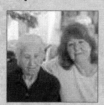

Susan realized that her mother, Estelle, could not manage a lot of stimulation. Estelle easily became agitated and confused, so Susan avoided taking her to places with large crowds or noisy environments. Susan discovered that soothing music calmed Estelle and used it to help her relax when she grew anxious and irritable. Establishing a routine with familiar faces in smaller groups has allowed Estelle to enjoy a better quality of life, despite the challenges caused by dementia with Lewy bodies.

Below are some important actions you can take to adjust to your new roles, be realistic about your situation, and care for yourself. See the "Resources" section for more information.

Educate Others About LBD

Most people, including many healthcare professionals, are not familiar with LBD. In particular, emergency room physicians and other hospital workers may not know that people with LBD are extremely sensitive to antipsychotic medications. Caregivers can educate healthcare professionals and others by:

- Informing hospital staff of the LBD diagnosis and medication sensitivities, and requesting that the person's neurologist be consulted before giving any drugs to control behavior problems.

- Sharing educational pamphlets and other materials with doctors, nurses, and other healthcare professionals who care for the person with LBD.

Materials are available from the Lewy Body Dementia Association (see the "Resources" section).

- Teaching family and friends about LBD so they can better understand your situation.

Prepare for Emergencies

People with LBD may experience sudden declines in functioning or unpredictable behaviors that can result in visits to the emergency room. Infections, pain, or other medical conditions often cause increased confusion or behavioral problems. Caregivers can prepare for emergencies by having available:

- a list of the person's medications and dosages
- a list of the person's health conditions, including allergies to medicines or foods
- copies of health insurance card(s)
- copies of healthcare advance directives, such as a living will
- contact information for doctors, family members, and friends

Adjust Expectations

You will likely experience a wide range of emotions as you care for the person with LBD. Sometimes, caregiving will feel loving and rewarding. Other times, it will lead to anger, impatience, resentment, or fatigue. You must recognize your strengths and limitations, especially in light of your past relationship with the person. Roles may change between a husband and wife or between a parent and adult children. Adjusting expectations can allow you to approach your new roles realistically and to seek help as needed.

People approach challenges at varied paces. Some people want to learn everything possible and be prepared for every scenario, while others manage best by taking one day at a time. Caring for someone with LBD requires a balance. On one hand, you should plan for the future. On the other hand, you may want to make each day count in personal ways and focus on creating enjoyable and meaningful moments.

Care for Yourself

As a caregiver, you play an essential role in the life of the person with LBD, so it is critical for you to maintain your own health and well-being. You may be at increased risk for poor sleep, depression, or illness as a result of your responsibilities. Watch for signs of physical or emotional fatigue such as irritability, withdrawal from friends and family, and changes in appetite or weight.

All caregivers need time away from caregiving responsibilities to maintain their well-being. Learn to accept help when it's offered and learn to ask family and friends for help. One option is professional respite care, which

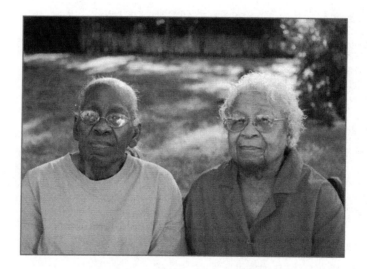

can be obtained through home care agencies and adult day programs. Similarly, friends or family can come to the home or take the person with LBD on an outing to give you a break.

Address Family Concerns

Not all family members may understand or accept LBD at the same time, and this can create conflict. Some adult children may deny that parents have a problem, while others may be supportive. It can take a while to learn new roles and responsibilities.

Family members who visit occasionally may not see the symptoms that primary caregivers see daily and may underestimate or minimize your responsibilities or stress. Professional counselors can help with family meetings or provide guidance on how families can work together to manage LBD.

Changing relationships

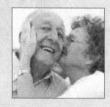

Diane's husband Jim was diagnosed with Lewy body dementia 2 years ago. Their son and daughter, who live across the country, thought that Diane was making too much of his illness. She asked them to fly out for a family meeting. A counselor who specializes in geriatrics gave the children helpful educational materials, and the family talked about the kind of emotional support Diane needs. They are on a better road to teamwork now.

Helping Children and Teens Cope with LBD

When someone has Lewy body dementia, it affects the whole family, including children and grandchildren. Children notice when something "doesn't seem right." Telling them in age-appropriate language that someone they know or love has been diagnosed with a brain disorder can help them make sense of the changes they see. Give them enough information to answer questions or provide explanations without overwhelming them.

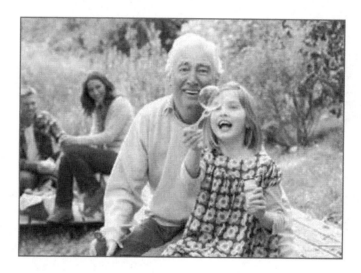

Children and teens may feel a loss of connection with the person with LBD who has problems with attention or alertness. They may also resent the loss of a parent caregiver's attention and may need special time with him or her. Look for signs of stress in children, such as poor grades at school, withdrawal from friendships, or unhealthy behaviors at home. Parents may want to notify teachers or counselors of the LBD diagnosis in the family so they can watch for changes in the young person that warrant attention.

Here are some other ways parents can help children and teens adjust to a family member with LBD:

- Help them keep up with normal activities such as sports, clubs, and other hobbies outside the home. Suggest ways for kids to engage with the relative with LBD through structured activities or play. For example, the child or teen can make a cup of tea for the person with LBD.

- Find online resources for older children and teens so they can learn about dementia and LBD. See the "Resources" section for more information.

It is important for families to make time for fun. Many challenges can be faced when they are balanced with enjoyable times. While LBD creates significant changes in family routines, children and teens will cope more effectively if the disorder becomes part of, but not all of, their lives.

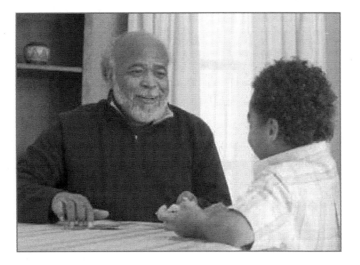

Research—The Road Ahead

There is a great deal to learn about LBD. At a basic level, why does alpha-synuclein accumulate into Lewy bodies, and how do Lewy bodies cause the symptoms of LBD? It is also of increasing interest to the Alzheimer's and Parkinson's disease research communities. LBD represents an important link between these other brain disorders, and research into one disease often contributes to better understanding of the others.

Many avenues of research focus on improving our understanding of LBD. Some researchers are working to identify the specific differences in the brain between dementia with Lewy bodies and Parkinson's disease dementia. Others are looking at the disease's underlying biology, genetics, and environmental risk 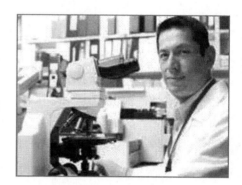 factors. Still other scientists are trying to identify biomarkers (biological indicators of disease), improve screening tests to aid diagnosis, and research new treatments.

Scientists hope that new knowledge about LBD will one day lead to more effective treatments and even ways to cure and prevent the disorder. Until then, researchers need volunteers with and without LBD for clinical studies.

To find out more about clinical trials, talk with a doctor or visit the National Institutes of Health Web site at *www.clinicaltrials.gov* and *www.nih.gov/health/clinicaltrials*.

Resources

Federal Government

National Institute on Aging
Alzheimer's Disease Education and Referral (ADEAR) Center
1-800-438-4380 (toll-free)
adear@nia.nih.gov
www.nia.nih.gov/alzheimers

National Institute of Neurological Disorders and Stroke
1-800-352-9424 (toll-free)
www.ninds.nih.gov

MedlinePlus
National Library of Medicine
www.medlineplus.gov
www.medlineplus.gov/spanish

General Information

Lewy Body Dementia Association
1-800-539-9767 (toll-free LBD Caregiver Link)
1-404-935-6444 (national office)
lbda@lbda.org
www.lbda.org

Michael J. Fox Foundation for Parkinson's Research
1-800-708-7644 (toll-free)
www.michaeljfox.org

National Parkinson Foundation
1-800-473-4636 (toll-free helpline)
contact@parkinson.org
www.parkinson.org

Parkinson's Disease Foundation
1-800-457-6676 (toll-free helpline)
info@pdf.org
www.pdf.org

Support Services and Resources

Eldercare Locator

This service of the U.S. Administration on Aging connects the public to community services for older adults and their families.

1-800-677-1116 (toll-free)

www.eldercare.gov

Family Caregiver Alliance

The Alliance provides information and referral, education, and other services to caregivers of people with chronic, disabling health conditions.

1-800-445-8106 (toll-free)

info@caregiver.org

www.caregiver.org

For Children and Teens

Although the following Alzheimer's organizations are not specific to Lewy body dementia, their dementia-related resources and networks may be helpful for children and teens.

ADEAR Center Resources for Children and Teens

www.nia.nih.gov/alzheimers/resources-children-and-teens-about-alzheimers-disease

Alzheimer's Association Kids & Teens

1-800-272-3900 (toll-free)

www.alz.org/living_with_alzheimers_just_for_kids_and_teens.asp

Alzheimer's Foundation of America (AFA) Teens

1-866-232-8484 (toll-free)

www.afateens.org

Diagnosis, Treatment, and Research

The Lewy Body Dementia Association (LBDA) maintains a list of its scientific and medical advisors. Many of these physicians see patients at their clinics or may make referrals to other specialists in your area. See *www.lbda.org/content/lbda-scientific-advisory-council-sac*. For general tips on finding a doctor, visit *www.lbda.org/content/finding-doctor-diagnose-and-treat-lbd*.

The Alzheimer's Disease Education and Referral Center maintains a list of research centers funded by the National Institute on Aging at NIH where you may find medical specialists in Lewy body dementia: *www.nia.nih.gov/alzheimers/alzheimers-disease-research-centers*.

The American Academy of Neurology has a "find a neurologist" page on its website: *http://patients.aan.com/findaneurologist*.

The American Association for Geriatric Psychiatry has a physician finder on its website: *http://gmhfonline.org*.

Acknowledgments

The National Institute on Aging and the National Institute of Neurological Disorders and Stroke thank the following people for their contributions to the vision and creation of this booklet:

Lisa Snyder, MSW, LCSW
Director, Quality of Life Programs
Shiley-Marcos Alzheimer's Disease Research Center
University of California, San Diego

Christina Gigliotti, PhD
Community Health Program Supervisor
Shiley-Marcos Alzheimer's Disease Research Center
University of California, San Diego

Angela Taylor
Director of Programs
Lewy Body Dementia Association

Scientific and Medical Reviewers from the LBDA Scientific Advisory Council

Douglas Galasko, MD
Co-Director, Shiley-Marcos Alzheimer's Disease Research Center
University of California, San Diego

Howard Hurtig, MD
Chair, Department of Neurology
Pennsylvania Hospital

James Leverenz, MD
Director, Cleveland Lou Ruvo Center for Brain Health-Neurological Institute

Caregiver Reviewers

Nancy Archibald
Kathleen Burr
Paul Smith
Joy Walker

The National Institute on Aging (NIA) and the National Institute of Neurological Disorders and Stroke (NINDS) are part of the National Institutes of Health, the nation's medical research agency—supporting scientific studies that turn discovery into health.

NIA leads the federal government effort conducting and supporting research on aging and the health and well-being of older people. NIA's Alzheimer's Disease Education and Referral (ADEAR) Center offers information and publications on dementia and caregiving for families, caregivers, and professionals.

NINDS is the nation's leading funder of research on the brain and nervous system. The NINDS mission is to reduce the burden of neurological disease.

For additional copies of this publication or further information, contact:

National Institute on Aging
Alzheimer's Disease Education and Referral Center
www.nia.nih.gov/alzheimers
1-800-438-4380

National Institute of Neurological Disorders and Stroke
www.ninds.nih.gov
1-800-352-9424

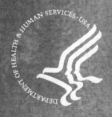
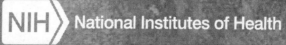

Publication No. 15-7907
September 2015

Made in the USA
Columbia, SC
15 November 2024

46618385R00026